I0101798

High Fructose Corn Poison

By Curtis R. Crim BA

All Rights Reserved
Copyright © 2009 by Curtis R. Crim BA
No part of this book may be reproduced or
transmitted in any form or by any means,
electronic or mechanical, including photocopying,
recording, or by any information
storage and retrieval system without permission
in writing from the author.

ISBN: 978-0-615-34292-4

Printed in the United States of America

First Printing

This book is lovingly dedicated to my
organic farm, and the Mother Nature there
who loves, teaches and nourishes my family.

TABLE OF CONTENTS

Preface:
"The purpose of this book"

The United States of America is not only one of the most powerful nations on the planet in terms of food production; it is also, like Egypt, one of the most powerful producers of food in human history.

What an irony then, that the food industry of the USA is now in a state of crisis. Most people are not aware of how bad the problem is, because the American advertising industry is so effective.

With the health of Americans in jeopardy, including that of our children and armed forces, and with the fact that we are facing the possibility of losing an entire generation, this crisis has now escalated to the point where public awareness of this disaster is essential.

The primary purpose of this book is to raise awareness of what I am calling the Great American Food Crisis. I will propose several solutions to this crisis, but the first step towards any solution at all is to bring this disaster to the attention of all Americans.

That American citizens should be made aware of this crisis is a necessity of emergency proportions, but how are we to address the issue that American food has become poison? This author hesitates to use the terminology and lexicon provided by the advertising industry.

They say that the pen is mightier than the sword, meaning that words (used to manipulate awareness, consciousness and people's way of thinking) are more powerful than military might. Many battles have been won on propaganda alone. I conclude that words are both tools and weapons, and since we are in a food emergency, it is important that we address the issue while choosing our words carefully.

I am going to use an analogy to illustrate why it would be a mistake to use the terminology provided by the enemy of the American public (the American food industry.) Imagine that you are a slave who is going to go into the arena to face a heavily armed, armored and experienced gladiator. You are given a gladius, and nothing else. You might think that the sword will help you survive the battle, but that was given to you for your execution.

The basic point is that it would be better to be able to choose your own armor and weapon, and better still if you could forge weapons to your own specifications, or have them custom made to fit this particular battle. Take your enemy's weapons and use them against him whenever possible, but never accept a weapon that is willingly provided you by your enemy.

So we now are going up against monsters as powerful as dragons, and the only weapons we have to use are words. Since this appears to be the case, I choose to forge my own lexicon and system of terminology in order to address the nationwide disaster we are now facing. The second purpose of this book is to introduce this new lexicon.

Third, I will address possible solutions to this problem, which will also help prepare humanity for 2012 (massive solar magma blast.) These solutions include approaches on the personal, communal and governmental levels.

In order to address an issue of this magnitude, it would be good to start from a common perspective.

Introduction: A Common Basis of Understanding

I became aware of the Great American Food Crisis after watching a set of documentaries, all of which I highly recommend. So that we can discuss the food disaster that America is facing, it will help considerably if you would continue your education by watching each of these documentaries, as I will also be referring to material in them in this text. I do not plan to present new information in this book, per se, so we will rely on these previous works to supply most of the supporting facts.

You can watch these in any order you like, but I highly recommend that you view each of them, before moving on to the next chapter. The following documentaries are all available from Netflix, and you can probably find them available in many video rental stores and on-line services: "King Corn", "Super Size Me", "Food Inc.", "Fast Food Nation" and "Killer at Large: Why Obesity is America's Greatest Threat".

Not only do I recommend that you see these documentary films, but I suggest that you consider each one a "must see" if you plan to eat or feed your family in modern-day America. Food is one of the essentials for survival, and the food you eat should be of great importance to you. If you plan to take your kids to a restaurant, it is important that you know what is really going into their bodies, because their future health is dependant upon proper nutrition when they are young. Because of this fact, and the fact that the "food" in America is now poison, one of the most relevant shows you will EVER see is "Food Inc."

The Americans who are aware of the America Food Crisis feel so strongly about this nation-wide disaster that many communities are now holding public showings of this movie. If you want to see it with friends and neighbors, contact your city hall and find out when the next showing will be. If they don't have it on the schedule, then request that they set it up. After public viewings of Food Inc. there is generally an open forum discussion about the problem and how to deal with it. As a responsible American citizen, you should see Food Inc. as soon as possible!

In addition, I advise that you supplement the material presented in Food Inc. with the other documentaries I am recommending. "King Corn" is an excellent presentation of the American corn industry, and shows in detail how many products and how much of our food supply come from corn. "Super

Size Me" illustrates in detail how quickly one can destroy one's internal organs by over-consuming High Fructose Corn Poison (HFCP.) "Killer at Large" shows what consuming HFCP is doing to the youth and armed forces of America. "Fast Food Nation" is a movie, not a documentary, but it is well worth watching. It addresses health risks of "junk food", and how fast food "restaurants" are an integral part of American culture.

 So get to it and watch these shows so that we all have a common basis of understanding of the Great American Food Crisis, then proceed to the next chapter.

Chapter 1: Forging a New Lexicon

The American advertising industry is expert in brain washing. The people who sell their advertising services to corporations also have no moral problem with lying in commercials, as well as employing dirty tactics like subliminal messages, innuendo and implication. When people watch a commercial, they get brainwashed on many levels simultaneously. When dealing with the Great American Food Crisis, it is necessary to address the role played by the advertising industry. They are word smiths with great psychological knowledge of human beings, and know exactly how to use words to brainwash the citizens of America.

Because of this, I cannot afford to fall into the trap of using the terminology they have invented and supplied as part of our demise. I will discuss the HFCP addiction epidemic using my newly proposed lexicon in order to AVOID the brainwashing the advertising industry has inherently programmed into their set of terms and phrases that have become part of the commercial American culture.

Normally, a glossary comes at the end of a book. Further, many of these terms have pretty obvious meanings. If I were to say, "That Coke is loaded with High Fructose Corn Poison.", you would know exactly what the meaning is without my having to explain it. However, a major goal of this book is to introduce a new set of terms and phrases to help focus awareness on the crisis in which we find ourselves, without submitting to the brainwashing of the advertising industry. Therefore an in-depth definition and explanation of each term and phrase is in order.

Of course, the terms and phrases which I am now inventing will, if adopted by the culture, be modified and permuted in various ways, and even take on new meanings. It is my goal to have as many people adopt my new terminology as possible, to give them a better chance of surviving the attacks on their consciousness by the advertising industry.

The New Great American Food Crisis
HFCP Lexicon

"High Fructose Corn Poison" – The term currently used, "High Fructose Corn Syrup", is dripping with the brain washing of the advertising industry, and it should be banned from food labels and replaced with this term.

The fact that they call it "syrup" implies strongly that it is food, when in fact it is refined to the point that it is actually a drug. It is as addictive as heroine and nicotine. HFCP is at least as destructive to human internal organs as ethyl alcohol. It is an incredibly dangerous drug that is used to addict people to fast junk while making the food industry obscenely wealthy. (Also, just for the conspiracy freaks out there, keep in mind that all fast junk saloons are owned by Coke and Pepsi, who are in turn owned by Exxon/Mobile and other OIL corporations! The same people who put a dictator in the White House are also the ones whom the dictator in turn put in control of the agencies protecting their victims from them! Well done!) HFCP is also currently America's largest export on an annual basis, in the form of Coke and other soft drink products. By substituting the word "poison" for the word "syrup", we accentuate the effects that HFCP has on human physiology. I would like congress to pass an amendment that would require a bright red sign with a skull and crossbones and the word "POISON" in various languages to be required, and to be prominently displayed on every product that contains HFCP. Of course, this is not going to happen because the corporations of the American food industry (this includes the oil and chemical corporations, by the way) have total control over the three main branches of the Federal Government of the USA, and most of the regulatory commissions as well. I believe that many people will object to the use of the word "poison" and insist that HFCP is not poison at all. I therefore need to clarify what food is and what poison is. Here is my personal test: Take some substance to be tested and get enough that you can eat nothing but that for a month. Example, get a few cases of broccoli. If you eat nothing but broccoli for an entire month, you might lose some excess weight, you might be stronger and smarter at the end of the month, but you won't be dead. Example, you repeat the same experiment and consume nothing but whisky for a month. You can have water during this experiment, but only H2O is allowed in addition to the substance under test. During the course of this second experiment, you will die. Ethyl alcohol is a poison, and you won't survive a month of nothing but whisky and water. Now, to the real issue: Example number 3: You get a couple of 5 gallon tins of High Fructose Corn Poison. You can eat that and water for a whole month, but that is all. You might live (slightly) longer than the person consuming nothing but whisky and water for a month, but you won't live much longer, and you won't survive the whole month. This is because HFCP is not food. It is poison and it is highly addictive, and it is in almost every food product available in

America in 2009. Given time, it will destroy your liver, pancreas, spleen and kidneys, not to mention what it will do to your arteries and cardiac muscle!

"Fast Junk" – For too long now, the American advertising industry has manipulated us with various phrases that *imply* meaning in order to brainwash people into spending their money on products that are not really food at all. "Food" from McDonald's, for instance, is really not food at all. It is not "Fast Food", and it is not "Junk Food". It simply isn't food of any kind. Therefore, the new term is "Fast Junk". It is appropriate not only because it is descriptive, but also because one use of the word "junk" is to refer to heroine (highly refined opium poppy sap), which is as addictive as high fructose corn poison. The stuff you buy at McDonald's or Burger King or Pizza Hut is fast (when you are lucky), and it certainly is JUNK (few people would deny that.) I have heard of people referring to high quality, low fat meat as brain food, or even cauliflower or broccoli, but NEVER a Big Mac. In fact, and I will elaborate on this later in this book, but when you eat Fast Junk, it actually reduces your higher brain functions such as memory, logic and cognitive thought. When I was a kid, they had actual Junk Food. It was food with a high carbohydrate content and very little nutritional value. But then when I was a kid, they didn't have genetically engineered High Fructose Corn Poison either. The McDonald's hamburger you buy today looks exactly like the one my Dad bought for us back in the 1960's, but the fast junk hamburger of today is nothing like it was forty or fifty years ago. The meat is manufactured in such a way as to make it much more dangerous these days; the ketchup is now loaded with genetically engineered HFCP.

"Fast Junk Saloon" – These are commonly known as "Fast Food Restaurants". Again, it is inappropriate to call McDonald's any kind of a restaurant. They don't serve food, they serve poison. We do have a cultural context for an establishment that sells recreationally consumed poison. We call it a "saloon", a "tavern" or a "bar". Some people will disagree that ethyl alcohol is poison, but it most literally is. At CSU alone, one or more students drink themselves to death once or twice a year, usually during the frat/sorority rush, or at the "Spring Fling". This happens when some idiot takes on the bet as to whether he can chug a quart of Tequila, and then fails to regurgitate prior to losing consciousness. I had a friend named Debbie who drank herself to death at a party at the young age of only thirteen. We can see clearly that consuming poison in moderate doses is part of American culture. So now look at McDonald's. People go there because they are addicted to highly refined genetically engineered High Fructose Corn Poison, a dangerous narcotic drug, not because they are hungry and need food. In fact, if your body is hungry and desperate for actual food, eating fast junk is one of the worst things you can do to your physiology! If after chopping a lot of wood in the forest, I come in and eat anything with HFCP in it, I will become nauseated and regurgitate. Poisoning the body when it needs nourishment frequently results in regurgitation. That is why you so often see puke in the parking lots of Fast Junk Saloons (and drinking establishments), but almost never see it in the parking lots of natural organic food restaurants. Poisoning the body is dangerous and destructive to one's health. That is why my new term for these establishments is "Fast Junk Saloons". This term focuses attention on the fact that they sell a poisonous narcotic drug, not nourishing food. The attempt here, as in all of these terms, is to strip away the layers of brainwashing that have been put in place by the American advertising industry.

"The Great American Food Crisis" – I find that more and more people these days are seeing the epidemic of obesity and diabetes in America as a serious problem. Although I agree, I think that the word "problem" is not sufficient to describe a situation where parents are being brainwashed into poisoning their own children, to the point were we could lose an entire generation of Americans. We are, my friends, in a crisis situation. It is an emergency. The goal of addressing this issue now is to prevent this situation from deteriorating into the Great American Food Disaster. More children now have early onset type two diabetes than ever before. America is now not only the fattest nation in the world, per capita, but it is also the fattest nation in human history. Our armed forces now lose more limbs and lives to obesity and diabetes (by far!) than they do to all forms of military combat combined! This situation doesn't just appear to be a problem to me; it appears to be a crisis: The Great American Food Crisis.

"Treason" – This is not a new word, but I wish to add another meaning to its list of definitions in the dictionary. One definition, of course, is the subversion of an executive election. The new meaning that I wish to add is what is now called "lobbying". The original meaning of lobbying was that a person who is concerned about an issue could approach their congressman in the lobby of congress during a break and bring their issue to the senator or representative's attention. What lobbying has become these days is multinational mega-corporations' bribing of congressmen with drugs, real estate, vehicles and money (and sex) to give the MMC's more and more power. This, obviously, is unfair to the American public, and is a direct attack on our system of politics. Because of this, it is treason, and the multinational mega corporations get away with it daily. This is why I think that American English should do away with the word "lobbying" altogether, and use the word "treason" in its place.

"MMC's" – This is just an acronym for Multinational Mega Corporations. In order to discuss the Great American Food Crisis, it is absolutely necessary that we put some awareness on these monsters of corporations. These metaphorical dragons are responsible for poisoning your children, and they include names like Coke, Pepsi Co., Tyson's and Monsanto. They are guilty of treason, have no morals at all, and have only one motivation: profit. I am tempted to go off on a rant here, but don't want to diverge from the central subject of this book: High Fructose Corn Poison. Therefore, if you want to know more about the dangers of MMC's and what the solutions to their existence might include, then please look for my upcoming book, "Corporateocracy." This book will examine what the form of the US Government is. It is not a Democracy, as

is constantly brainwashed into most
American citizens. We live in a society
where the Federal Government is controlled
by and is of, by, and for the MMC's, and
against the American people. That's not a
democracy, it is a Corporateocracy.

Chapter 2: A Cultural Disaster: The Great American Food Crisis

One thing that is so frustrating about HFCP is that it is hidden in America's food supply. You would literally be shocked if you knew each and every product it is in. This is one of the reasons that it is so easy to get addicted to the stuff; frequently, people don't even know that they are eating it!

Sure, most people know that virtually all soda pop contains it in large quantities, as does ketchup, Hershey's chocolate syrup and most ice creams. But they sneak it into products where one would not expect it unless one reads the ingredients list. Here is an example (you can verify this for yourself): Swanson's has a vegetarian broth that one might expect to be healthy just because it is advertised as being vegetarian. After all, vegetarians are generally health and health-food oriented, and not as likely to eat fast junk. Obviously, they want to eat food that doesn't harm their physiology. However, Swanson's Vegetarian Broth has a label that clearly states in the Ingredients section that it contains HFCP. So this apparently innocuous food actually contains a powerful and highly addictive poisonous drug.

The effects that HFCP has on the system are devastating, but this substance is dangerous and destructive to our culture on a psychological level as well. Even intelligent well educated health specialists sometimes come under its insidious spell. Here is a little real-life example. In college, I worked for several vegetarian and natural-food oriented restaurants and food services. These restaurants mostly catered to the local vegetarian population associated with the local university. One very nice woman I worked for ran a successful restaurant that made delicious food that was highly appealing to the local vegans. Her customers were primarily vegetarians who seek out natural and organic food, and she is well educated in how to produce proper healthy food. Obviously, I am not going to mention her name so as not to cause embarrassment. I recently ran into her in the local grocery store (a chain store, not a health-food grocery.) She was still very sweet and it was nice to visit with her, but she had a shopping cart with several cases of coca-cola in it, and she had gained about 70 LBS since we had worked together. She explained that she is addicted to it, and could not control the urge to drink it. I was surprised, because I felt that she was someone who would know better than to destroy her physiology with poison. The advertising and food industries in America were clever enough to get to her. I guess she is just one more victim of these monsters. How sad.

Here is another example: My sister tries to feed her family the best, most healthy food available anywhere. She will actually pay over $10 a pound for carrots just to get the ones that are not only organic but also certified non-genetically engineered! Not only does her family eat only vegetarian food products, they also eat some of the most natural and healthy food available. However, she doesn't protect her family from HFCP with 100% effectiveness. At Halloween, her kids are allowed to gorge on commercially produced candy, most of which contains HFCP. Her son said that they occasionally drink a soft drink, even though they know that it contains HFCP. My brother in law told me that they occasionally order pizza from Pizza Hut, and that pizza contains HFCP in the crust as well as the sauce! The point being that even a woman trying her hardest to protect her family from this poison can fail due to the effective strategies employed by the American advertising and food industries.

I have, like most Americans, also been addicted to High Fructose Corn Poison. My drug of choice is the Pizza Hut Meatlover's on the thin and crispy crust. The last time I ordered this product I had it made with the bean sauce (used on the taco pizza) instead of the red sauce, so as to avoid the majority of the HFCP. I went into The Hut about a month ago, and ordered the wings. I got some ranch and blue cheese with them for dipping. When I got home, I read the ingredients on the ranch and blue cheese dressings, and they BOTH contained HFCP! I immediately threw the stuff out. I know that people who are addicted to HFCP can't live a day without it, but it makes me sick to consume it in even small quantities. I have always loved pizza, and Pizza Hut makes my favorite pizza that is available locally. However, I now throw the coupons away. I have not gone near a fast junk saloon since then, and feed myself by cooking healthy natural food, much of which I grow myself.

It is, of course, very hard to wean yourself off of fast junk emotionally. It helps to go to McDonald's and eat a healthy meal or two before saying goodbye forever. If you try really hard, you can get a healthy meal almost anywhere, even at McDonald's! Try this experiment in self-control: Go to McDonalds and order a classic grilled chicken sandwich minus the mayo (which is awful at McD's anyway) and an ice water. When you sit down, open up the sandwich and eat the lettuce, the tomato and the chicken breast. Save the bun and give it to your dog, who will love you for it. You have now had a decent healthy meal at McDonald's fast junk saloon, which is almost a contradiction by definition. You get to have that McDonald's feeling (for emotional weaning purposes), and at the same time have not poisoned yourself with HFCP. Just remember when you are in there that you cannot have ketchup, the shakes, any soft drink or any bun type product. If you wish, you can have some fries which are only junk food, not fast junk, but I don't recommend them for anyone on a diet, and only rarely for anyone not on a diet.

One aspect of this food crisis is that the fast junk saloons are so well integrated into American culture. Their food, appearance and advertisements have all become part of the American identity. It is hard to envision America without all of the fast junk. Whether we enjoy eating McDonald's food or not, and regardless of whether we allow ourselves to enjoy a Coca Cola, these products are part of our cultural identity. The main reason for this is the outstanding effectiveness of the American advertising industry.

Chapter 3: The Advertising Industry:
Selling Poison and Making You Swallow It

The American advertising industry is more than the evil I have made it out to be. It has been part of our culture for hundreds of years. It has helped to form the culture we see around us, and in no small way.

I was surprised to find out that Rudolph the Red Nosed reindeer was not made into a cartoon and part of our Christmas mythos after being originally written as a charming story for children. Rather, this character was invented by someone working for Wards, and it was invented specifically and exclusively as an advertising mechanism! It was a long time ago, so the origins of Rudolph have been forgotten, and he has become integrated into our Christmas mythology.

This is how powerful the advertising industry is. Someone can get an idea for a slogan or advertising mechanism like Rudolph, and change a culture for all time. How many slogans, even from decades ago can you remember? "It's the real thing!", "A Pepsi Generation", "Where's the beef?" quickly jump into my head, as well as tunes and lyrics from various commercials. The power of advertisement is awesome.

The power of the advertisement industry is even greater. This power is sadly and immorally abused. I personally consider all advertisement to be offensive, but the advertising industry employs evil tactics to manipulate and brainwash potential customers. It is possible to simply state the virtues of a product or service, and make it seem attractive by describing how good it is, but that is not good enough for the advertising industry that sees and takes advantage of many more subtle mechanisms to confuse, manipulate, brainwash and "dumb down" the public.

One such mechanism is the use of implications. Outright lies are okay, like "Women will notice you if you use Axe for men!" Sure, that sounds, good, but if women don't notice you anyway, wearing smelly crap will not change the situation at all. However, implying something that is not true is much more powerful that stating it outright. If one has to come to a conclusion on his own based on an implication, he is much more likely to believe it.

Subliminal mechanisms are also used constantly. These come in the form of hidden text and images, and also subtle placement of images that are obvious, and are designed to affect the psyche on a sub-conscious level. One example is the use of covertly sexual images that are designed to affect watchers without them being aware of it.

Have you ever seen a commercial that was so far from reality that it appeared to be completely retarded to you? This is intentional. Exposing people to retarded scenarios tends to decrease their intelligence, both their actual knowledge and their ability to learn. I personally am offended when I have such retardation presented to me, but I have a DVR and rarely expose myself to commercials. I call it "mental hygiene". The reason the advertisement industry uses commercials to retard the watcher is that it is easier to get people to believe their lies and be subjugated by their manipulation if they are stupid. Commercials effectively make people more stupid. They just want your money, but if you are smart, you will never watch a commercial for any reason. My ex-wife loved commercials, and would weep when the kid only had two cavities, but she is also one of the stupidest people I have ever had the displeasure of knowing.

Manipulation is one of the most powerful mechanisms in the arsenal of the advertising industry, which they use against their enemy, the American public. The job of the MMC's and the advertising industry is to control the American public, and sell them a product: the American culture. But their version of the American culture is not comprehensive. In fact, that version of the American culture is materialistic, and lacking in true value. The American advertising industries' version of the American culture doesn't include people like Michael Moore, nor hermits who live without their crappy culture at all, or people who refuse to buy their lies and only eat food that they raise with their own hands. It doesn't include people who free range their livestock and butcher it by hand and provide healthy locally raised food to the local grocery stores. Their version of the American culture doesn't include people like me who think every word out of the advertising industry is a lie. Their version doesn't include the Amish, the Mennonites, the Transcendental Meditation community or any subculture that refuses to accept their commercialized, packaged version of American culture. My point is that their goal is to sell you their version of the American culture, but it is nowhere near a comprehensive vision of the actual real American culture that exists in this country right now. The advertising

29

industry does have a right to contribute to American culture; they do NOT have the right to DICTATE American culture!

Another very evil practice of the advertising industry is demographic targeting. You see this all of the time. McDonald's was clearly doing this in recent years. I saw a McDonald's commercial that showed African-Americans going to McDonald's and finding Utopia. They threw in a hip-hop/rap fusion musical theme in the background, and the lyrics and slogans were set to a beat appropriate for rap.

One of the sad realities is that the WORST food available in America is very inexpensive. The poor can only afford to eat (and feed their families) fast junk, crap and poison. Historically, the poor have always been the demographic in society to be exploited by all of the other classes, but here in America, the worst abuse of demographic targeting is the abuse of American children. The way children are targeted and brainwashed is heinously evil, mostly because they are so gullible and therefore not equipped to know when they are being lied to. It should be illegal, but the advertising industry are also such effective lobbyists (therefore, traitors), that they forced congress to allow them to victimize children. FOR SHAME! For this reason alone, the advertisers who are engaging in this practice should be tortured, salted and quartered for their treason against humanity, not just their treason against the American people.

Fast junk is love. At least, that is the way it is portrayed by the advertising industry. If you watch McDonald's commercials carefully, you will see how they are selling fast junk, but they are advertising love to the children who see their commercials. Every parent in America (or nearly so) knows that if you really want to make your child happy, you take them to McDonald's, right? They could easily just say that their food is tasty, but instead they manipulate the feelings of their audience by advertising good feelings, not good food. Most kids want very much to be loved, so they are very susceptible to this kind of advertisement. It is also part of our culture (forced upon us by the MMC's) that it is normal to be lied to and manipulated by commercials, and many people don't ever understand that they are being lied to in commercials. The MMC's and the advertising industry have made being victimized by the advertising industry a "normal" and accepted aspect of life in America. Children are not generally taught that what they see in commercials (and on the news) is just flat out lies, dishonesty and the distortion of actual reality. In other words, your children would be safer if you just let them know that they are being lied to. Instead, most parents let themselves be manipulated by their brainwashed children, and take the family out to a nice meal of poison at McDonalds. Then they are surprised when their 300 pound twelve year old has to have her feet amputated because she has diabetes from eating Heinz ketchup and drinking Pepsi Cola.

Most of advertising is a lie in one way or another. Here is an example of the dishonesty of the advertising industry: Just a few days ago I was in Wal-Mart (shameful, I know, but the small stores were all put out of business, and Wal-Mart is the only place to shop for most non-grocery items) and I saw a large display of Coke products. One product, a new version of Cherry 7-Up, had a label that caught my eye. It said on the label that it had anti-oxidants, which help fight cancer, and had a label that implies that it is natural and healthy. I couldn't believe it! I know this stuff to be some of the most toxic and addictive poison in the world, so I read the label. The second ingredient on the list was HFCP! So here they were advertising that this product is "healthy" for you, and in fact the second ingredient is poison! It is an unbelievable state of things, but the depth of the evil of the advertising

industry I will discuss in my next book,
Corporateocracy (releasing soon.)

Chapter 4: Taking Poison: An American Tradition

One of the most exceptionally stupid statements I have ever heard was said by my mother. I said that it is normal to consume poison in our culture, and she said, "But people don't take poison!" I was so surprised at her lack of awareness that I was left speechless for several moments, which is very rare for me. Dozens of thoughts and images started dancing through my brain, including memories of advertisements for Captain Morgan's and Corona Mexican beer.

I thought about a manager I once had when I was working for the corporations who once told me, "I don't do drugs." I knew him to have a drink after work, coffee in the morning, Coke during the day and a cigarette break at every opportunity. Again, it was such an ignorant thing to say that I had no idea how to form a though that would be appropriate to speak aloud at the time.

Let's examine just what we know about Mr. "I Don't Do Drugs": He consumes large amounts of caffeine in his morning coffee and in the Coke as well. Caffeine is an amphetamine, in the same chemical category as Crank (crystal Methedrine, aka methamphetamine), so he has that category of recreational drugs covered. He gets plenty of narcotics, because he is consuming both nicotine and HFCP, an equally dangerous and addictive narcotic, so that category of recreational drugs is also covered in his daily diet. He is drinking alcohol, which is a downer, although not a barbiturate, is still poison that can kill you quickly, and is well known to be addictive.

I think that the only category of recreational drugs that Mr. "I Don't Do Drugs" DOESN'T have covered is hallucinogens! LOL! What a freaking jackass! But then, he is brainwashed like 80% of all Americans. The advertising industry, if you actually believe their lies, dictates to retarded American citizens what is and what is not a "drug". HFCP is as addictive as heroine and nicotine. It is as *refined* as heroine as well. It is as destructive as any drug that is taken recreationally in our culture, and if you are really REALLY stupid or brainwashed, then you will actually consume products like Coke, Pepsi and Heinz ketchup.

America has bars, taverns and saloons where adults can go and buy beverages that include ethyl alcohol as an ingredient. Frequently, one can also smoke commercial cigarettes in these establishments. You can order a "Roman Coke" that contains ethyl alcohol, caffeine and HFCP all in the same beverage! That gives you three categories of recreational drugs at one time, and you can order this drink in almost any bar in America! Wheeeeee!

America has also had a strong tradition of consuming illegal recreational drugs. Further, poisonous substances are sometimes consumed in religious rites and vision quests.

This is not only true of the current day American culture, but it has been true of cultures all over the world going back at least ten thousand years.

Putting all of these facts together, one can see that consuming poison is and always has been part of our culture, since long before America existed.

To suggest that people don't intentionally consume poison is absurd. It has always been part of human culture. The difference now is that they are addicting people to dangerous narcotic substances without the knowledge of the victim. If these products were properly labeled, and people could make a conscious decision for themselves and for their families, then they could take responsibility for their decision to partake of a poison, rather than having it forced upon them unknowingly.

Chapter 5: Solutions: Personal, Community, And Government

Obviously, we can just boycott, burn down and destroy all of the fast junk products. The advertising and food industries are so integrated into our culture, our lives and our economy, that they can't just be thrown away over night.

On the other hand, considering the threat of the American Food Crisis, we must consider ourselves obligated to consider possible solutions, even if they are long term in nature.

I suggest that a disaster of this magnitude must be approached on multiple levels, including that of the individual/family, the community and the government. These are big subjects, so I am dedicating the next three chapters to these.

Keep in mind that many approaches and solutions are ones that I will not think of myself. Think of yourself as part of the solution to this crisis. My solutions are only suggestions, and I strongly support the idea of people getting together to come up with solutions of their own. After all, they only have their children to lose if they don't.

Chapter 6:
An Individual Solution:
I'm Not Going to Eat Their
Poison Anymore!

I understand that it is not easy to break an addiction. I have known a few friends who had enough good character and will power to break bad addictions like nicotine. Weaning yourself off of HFCP is a similar experience.

When a person is addicted to a highly refined narcotic substance like HFCP, he is likely to do anything to get it. Trying to break such an addiction is also one of the most horrible feelings that a person can experience. It is understood that this is a difficult thing to do, and that a person can go through a living hell trying to stop a habit like drinking Pepsi or Coke. However, if you are to save your internal organs, your habit must be stopped.

I perform very physically strenuous tasks on my farm, and by the time lunchtime comes around, I am frequently starving for a meal! If at that time I feed by body fast junk, I will feel physically ill, nauseated, tired and mentally drained. The genetically engineered HFCP has the secondary effect of making a person feel complacent and conformistic, and decreasing the brain's ability to perform higher cognitive functions such as logic and reasoning. In other words, fast junk actually makes you increasingly stupid over time. As you lose your intelligence, you are more susceptible to advertisements and brainwashing, in which case you will probably go out and consume more fast junk. If you can manage to break your HFCP addiction, you will find that fast junk is no longer appealing. Real, natural food is much better tasting anyway.

If on the other hand I come in exhausted and eat locally raised, free range, locally slaughtered meat with a low carbohydrate, low fat, low cholesterol vegetable like broccoli, I will shortly feel stronger and good inside. I will feel more powerful, more energetic and more intelligent! Better yet, when one eats food that one grew organically with his own hands, one can also feel a flow of spiritual energy from Mother Nature and the land upon which he lives. I know that non-spiritual people cannot understand that statement, but growing and eating your own food makes you closer to your land, the land that you love, and the land who loves you in return.

Remember that Mother Nature is a real, actual person, and she has made it clear that she actually NEEDS our love. She does not need our neglect, and she does not need our abuse. Would you hit your mother in the face? I hope not. I want the MMC's to STOP HITTING MOTHER NATURE IN THE FACE!

On a personal level, you can also care for your land with love. Use natural pesticides and don't be a customer of the American agri-business industry. Have the morals to NOT do business with Monsanto, and not use genetically engineered seeds or livestock. Understand that if you really love Mother Nature, and I mean not just with your heart, but more specifically with your ACTIONS, then Mother Nature will support you and make you stronger, healthier and smarter. I truly believe that loving the natural spirit of my land has helped me gain the wisdom and intelligence to write this book.

Speaking of being intelligent, learn to read the ingredients on foods that you buy in the store. You wouldn't BELIEVE the various products that end up being pumped with HFCP, products that don't seem to be an appropriate product to put that drug into. It is often put in bread products to "make them taste better", but I think it is really to help addict you to their drug, as so many people eat bread. HFCP is added to most salad dressings, almost all candy and ice cream products, ketchup, most commercially produced soups, and almost all processed meats (like hot dogs.)

Learn a defensive strategic approach to shopping in an American grocery store. Keep in mind that a large majority of processed foods (including Kraft Stovetop Stuffing) contain HFCP. Most isles in the grocery store should be avoided completely, like the cereal isle and the soda pop isle. In fact, most of the isles in the center of the store contain a majority of the processed foods, and you are generally safer going to specific departments where actual food is sold, like the produce section, the meat department, the organic foods department and the dairy department, for example. When you are at the meat department, again avoid processed meats generally. Look for locally raised meat, like the beef from the Amana colonies, which is locally ranged and raised and butchered by hand, so it is some of the best meat you can get anywhere, and it is delicious as well. It is also low in carbohydrates, and completely free of HFCP.

Food you cook yourself is always better than food that has been prepared before purchase. One problem in modern American society is that few people have time to cook at the times they are hungry and need a meal. I try to run a business and a farm at the same time, and take care of my kids, all alone. I certainly don't have time to cook for myself in the middle of the day! I schedule days in the summer and fall to harvest vegetables and cook and preserve food, and can and freeze as much as I am able. On the days that I don't have time to cook, I pull a container of Acorn squash soup or some Thai beef and broccoli out of the freezer and throw that in the microwave oven. I get a delicious, organic, healthy meal in about as much time as it would take someone to go through the fast junk drive-through, so I don't have to sacrifice my schedule to get excellent, healthy, low-cost food. Ultimately, every individual just has to come to the attitude on their own that they are just not going to consume commercial fast junk anymore! Do it for yourself, your family and the people who love you.

Learn to practice mental hygiene. Every time you see a commercial of any kind, whether it is a billboard, an email spam, a TV commercial or a radio commercial, remind yourself that it is a lie, and that they are trying to manipulate you and brainwash you. Try to limit your exposure to the American culture as it is spun by the advertising industry. Be suspicious of companies and corporations, be VERY suspicious of MMC's, and keep a careful eye on religions and governments. I believe that the current world has become very dangerous. I recommend that everyone actually adopt a suspicious and even paranoid attitude towards all human culture.

On the other hand, culture can also provide some of the possible solutions to the Great American Food Crisis, such as communities working together towards the common goal of a sustainable human presence on our little globe.

Chapter 7: Communities Providing a Solution

Local communities all over America are becoming alarmed by the quickly escalating American Food Crisis. Obesity and obesity related diseases like diabetes are now the leading causes of death in America in general, in American children, and in the American armed forces. Drinking Pepsi and Coke products is killing America. Something HAS to be done!

Food Inc. was recently shown at a public forum locally and a discussion was held afterwards, and public awareness of this national disaster was raised. Raising awareness of this crisis is one of the most important roles of local communities, but it is far from the only thing that people working together locally can do.

One marvelous service that is found in many communities is a farmer's market. These are awesome because you can get safely produced, locally produced, healthy, natural, organic and often non-genetically engineered foods. Fairfield, Iowa has a farmer's market, but they are only open during the warm months of the year. I hope that in the future communities will build large Morton buildings that are heated for comfort in winter where the local farmer's market can run all year, and every day rather than just on the weekends. If the vendor's pay a fee to the market, that money can be put towards building a mega greenhouse for the community that is propane heated and runs year-around. That way, more local healthy food could be produced and made available all of the time.

These local changes are also going to take time, but America doesn't have a lot of time. The crisis is growing too quickly to give us the luxury of time. The American culture has to adapt in order to survive. With awareness, the adoption of a more enlightened attitude can lead to better practices. It is more fun and healthy to grow and cook one's own food anyway, and it is better for the environment than the abuse of modern American agri-business. One can actually get a spiritual feeling from eating food one grew one's self. I have never heard of anyone claiming to have had a genuine spiritual feeling from eating McDonald's fast junk. The artificial, commercialized environment of a McDonald's fast junk saloon is the exact opposite of the beauty one sees in nature.

Although the contribution of local communities will be essential in combating the HFCP addiction epidemic, local, state and federal governments also have a role to play.

Chapter 8: Government Responsibility for the People

The American advertising and food industries are huge, and enormously powerful. Heinz was once involved in a plot with the W's grandfather to depose FDR. It failed, but they got away with treason with no penalty at all. The MMC's are way too powerful, and they are also completely in control of the USA Federal Government. This is very sad, as I liked the notion of the USA as a Democracy.

Frankly, these days I find the local, city, county and state governments more reliable, regardless of where you live in the USA.

Regardless of the level of government, one of the most important and helpful efforts that the government can make is to make the public aware of the American National Food Crisis. A budget for food crisis and HFCP awareness could be established, and flyers could be mailed to residential addresses. The government could put commercials on TV to make people aware of the HFCP addiction epidemic.

The government could also take a different approach to feeding the armed forces. You have certainly heard about a MASH unit (Mobile Army Surgical Hospital.) They could make mobile greenhouses that could produce healthy food for the troops and not murder them with HFCP. I understand that the American MMC's have 100% control over our Federal Government, and that they make a HUGE profit every year murdering our soldiers and our children, but common sense would dictate that the health and welfare of our armed forces should be a high priority for the Federal government.

The executive and legislative branches of the federal government could work together to establish legislation that would help to protect the consumer, like the signs I suggested that label foods containing the dangerous evil drug HFCP as "Poison" to keep retarded people informed about the dangers of such fast junk.

These branches of government could also appoint a regulatory commission specifically to protect the American people from being victimized by evil, murdering monsters like Coke, Pepsi, McDonalds, Tyson's, Pizza Hut, Heinz, Hershey, etc. It would in design be much like the FDA, but not the FDA because they are controlled by the monsters that lie to you and brainwash you into poisoning your children to death. It would be more like a consumer protection agency, call it the CPA, for instance, and their job would be to assure that companies are fully truthful on their labels, which currently is NOT the case. I read a lot of labels these days, and they lie on a frequent basis.

It would be helpful if the Center for Disease Control would issue a statement nationally to make the American public aware of the National Food Crisis, but I assume that they are not concerned with the health of the American public.

Our new esteemed President could declare a state of national emergency until the Great American Food Crisis is resolved, but I believe that he is busy applying himself to far more MODERATE issues, like the lack of an American primary education system or the lack of a sane socialized medical system. Surely, these are important issues, but they are not a crisis. The top killer of Americans on an annual basis is now HFCP and the massive epidemic of addiction to this powerful narcotic drug. I might be completely out of line, but I would think that the top killer of American people annually would be of concern to any president who is not a puppet of the MMC's. But who knows, it's not as though his first term is up yet.

Chapter 9: Envisioning the Future

I see great wisdom in the adaptation of the American culture to create new healthy food supplies, but it isn't as if we want American agri-business to die over night. In fact, it isn't ever necessary.

We are discussing very big corporations, and they have think tanks of their own. If they were to see into the future and understand that change is necessary, they could have the vision to capitalize on the concept of doing well by doing good, or more specifically make a comfortable profit producing good organic food instead of fast junk. If I were to make recommendations to Monsanto (as though they would listen to me!) I would suggest that they retire large corn and soybean fields near cities and towns, and build enormous greenhouses that would then product organic food to be sold at the local town/city. I would suggest that they go to the higher-cost method of producing meat by free-range rather than corn-fed and corralled. A smart corporation is always prepared and willing to adapt to the current and constantly changing culture.

Monsanto, for example, is very powerful. In a brilliant act of treason against the USA, creation and God, they were able to not only lobby but bribe many Republican senators to pass a bill that gave them power that only a God should have. They have altered the structure of DNA itself, and that is not a small accomplishment. They have taken over the agency that was created to protect their victims from them. This is a beautiful illustration of the power of money and corruption.

Although I do question the wisdom of the practice of genetic engineering, I don't mean to imply that we should abandon all advanced human technology. I actually like computers, and think that if properly employed, computers can help us produce healthy organic food. Purely automated greenhouses are known to be less productive than ones that are tended manually, but I envision an advanced computer with artificial intelligence that can monitor security and also internal environmental conditions, as well as be able to make decisions and control the temperature, air flow, light spectrum and interval and plant nutrient levels. I would then supplement the AI with my own skill set, and together we could produce huge amounts of excellent food with a minimum of effort and time on my part. Perhaps even a robot that pulls weeds would be of great assistance! I like the idea of having a very advanced computer, and at the same time own a wood-burning cook stove to heat my home and cook organic food produced on my own farm. Maybe old and new human technology can be combined in a harmonious way so as to get the best of both worlds – the connection with nature of the old with the convenience and power of the new.

I put in surveillance systems for security, and they have proven to be the best way for me to keep an eye on my kids! If you care about something and want to nourish it, then keep your attention on it. With a controlled heart and mind, one can protect one's own universe and the people in it from the poison of the American culture as spun by the advertisement industry, and as served up by the American food industry.

I know that not all of my vision for the future and suggested solutions to the Great American Food Crisis are realistic. For one thing, we don't live in a Democracy where we get to choose leaders who look out for our best interests. We live in a Corporateocracy where we get the illusion of voting for our leaders, where *actually* our

government is of, for, and by the
Multinational Mega Corporations who
control our economy, our food supply, our
bodies and our minds. The fact that the
MMC's are now in iron-clad control of the
USA Federal Government appears to me to
be a disaster of mythic proportions, so I plan
to dedicate my next book, Corporateocracy,
to this subject, while others are addressing
artificial matters, such as a war illegally
declared by an illegal dictator.

Conclusion: Summary and Call to Arms

Every day, more and more Americans are becoming aware that we are in a National Food Crisis. Ironically, the Federal Government so far has refused to acknowledge the disaster that our nation is facing. Not only has a national state of emergency not been declared (so far), but the government seems to be ignoring the situation COMPLETELY and allowing the American food industry to (metaphorically) butcher American citizens by the millions while the advertising industry spins their lies and brainwashing. The situation is not only an emergency; it is also nothing less than *pathetic*.

Historically, the rich have always victimized the poor in all cultures ever since the dawn of civilization. Perhaps this practice goes back to the beginning of human culture itself. The American food industry has once again managed to make only poisonous food available to the poor, who lose their lives eating junk so the white male aristocrats can become even more obese financially.

My father, were he still alive, might remind me to examine this crisis from a haptic point of view, as opposed to my more Marxist perspective. Haptics refers to the sense of touch, and I think most people are (personally) aware of the haptics of being addicted to a dangerous, evil narcotic drug such as HFCP. Many Americans are aware of the haptic feedback experienced when trying to break an addiction to cigarettes, coffee, alcohol, a recreational drug like coke, crack or heroine or the most evil narcotic of all: HFCP. It's like when you are dieting, and you are starving yourself because you are desperate to go down another pound. It is the worst feeling you can possibly imagine, both inside and on the surface of your body. The only thing worse than that feeling is experiencing withdrawal from a narcotic drug to which you have become addicted.

On the other hand, if you don't break your addiction to HFCP your addiction will probably kill you. By allowing your family to consume HFCP, you are allowing it to kill them as well. I conclude that a majority of America is addicted to a narcotic substance and are not even aware of it.

A couple of days ago I went to a convenience store to get some milk for a soup I was making. Ahead of me was a farmer (clearly, from his complexion and attire) who was buying some tater tots from their hot section, a bag of generic potato chips and a Pepsi. To most people, this would appear to be a very normal scene. To me, it was a vision of the whole cycle of food insanity that has this nation in its grips. This guy almost certainly buys genetically engineered seed from Monsanto, and then sells them to corporations who make ketchup and poison like the Pepsi he was buying to drink himself! Not to mention the fact that everything he was buying was carbohydrates, which are junk food at the best! I saw a man who has no clue as to the Food Crisis America is now facing, a man who has no idea how dangerous HFCP is, and a man who has no idea what his highly ironic role in the insanity is! He just seemed very naïve and uninformed. I guess you don't learn much when you sit on a tractor all day!

The one thing that is clear is that something has to be done. The more people you can get to eat healthy food, the more people will be able to think clearly and organize a highly logical and effective defense against the enemies of the American people, the MMC's.

Whether your part is great or small, every person can make some difference in trying to save not only America but the entire world from the monster that the food industry has become. If you just boycott the fast junk saloons, or can give up Coke, then you have made a difference. Do it for yourself, if you cannot do it for your family and the people who love you. If you can be instrumental in raising community awareness of the crisis, then you have made a difference. If you just want to raise and sell organic vegetables at your local farmer's market, then you can also make an important difference in the lives of other families. It is important that you take the personal responsibility to make a difference in some way, even if it is small. If we all use our brains, we can work together to beat this thing. Greed is an evil that attacks our culture on many levels, but we cannot afford to let it poison our food supply or we are all doomed!

www.ingramcontent.com/pod-product-compliance
Lightning Source LLC
Chambersburg PA
CBHW060641280326
41933CB00012B/2104